The First-Time Cruiser's Guide to Staying Healthy

How to Eat, Sleep, Reduce Stress, Stay Hydrated and Exercise to Stay Healthy While Traveling on the High Seas

RON KNESS

Contents

Disclaimer

This publication is for informational purposes only and is not intended as medical advice. Medical advice should always be obtained from a qualified medical professional for any health conditions or symptoms associated with them.

Every possible effort has been made in preparing and researching this material. We make no warranties with respect to the accuracy, applicability of its contents or any omissions.

See your healthcare professional before starting any diet or exercise program!

Introduction

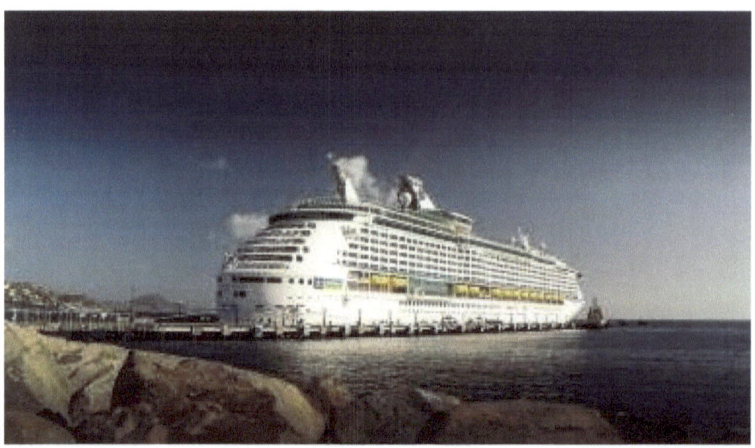

Traveling is stressful ... period. Couple that with sleeping in a different bed, eating different food, not exercising properly, not drinking enough water, being exposed to different germs and viruses, and you have a recipe for getting sick while on a cruise. However, there are several things you can do to stay healthy and enjoy yourself, instead of sitting in your ship cabin miserable and trying to get well.

As a veteran of almost 20 cruises, I have noticed three things initially that usually catch up to people after about Day 3 when on a cruise vacation: too much sun, too little sleep and too much alcohol.

Too Much Sun

Cruise ships make it easy to relax in a lounger beside one of many pools on a ship. However, in many cases, the place you sit will be out in full sun.

While sitting there soaking up the warmth (and getting your vitamin D) is inviting, especially if this is your getaway from the cold and snow, too much exposure to El Sol can result in dehydration, overheating, and if not careful, sunburn.

I'm not saying to not enjoy the sun, but do it smartly. First, use plenty of sunscreen – at least a SPF 30 or higher. Follow the manufacture's recommendation as far as when to apply. Some say 15 minutes before exposure while others may be as long as 30 minutes. And heed the reapply instructions too; some are good up to 80 minutes, but If you are in and out of the pool, you may have to reapply sooner.

Second, avoid the time of day when the sun is strongest. Mornings until about 10am and again after 2pm will usually keep you out of the hottest part of the day in most localities.

Too Little Sleep

On most of the ships, there is something going on until the wee hours of the morning every day. You are there to have fun and want to experience as much as you can, however, pace yourself. It is not an environment your body is used to and after a couple of days of partying, it is going to tell you to slow down. Ensure you are getting at least 7 to 8 hours of sleep per night. If that means getting in a nap or two during the day, then so be it.

Too Much Alcohol

So you are exposing your pale skin to more sun each day than you may normally see in a week or more and partying until all hours of the night. During each of these activities, you are more than likely consuming alcoholic drinks too.

However this again is more than likely not what you do at home on a regular basis, so this is all foreign to your body. Without offsetting the drying effects of the alcohol with water, along with water lost from sweat while sunning, it is easy to become dehydrated.

Let's look at the symptoms, effects and how to stay hydrated while on a cruise.

Staying Hydrated

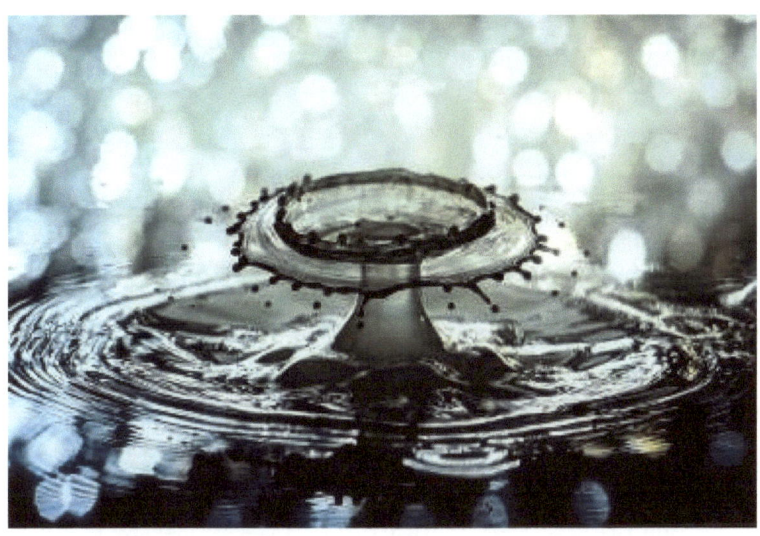

If you do not drink enough water, sweat too much, or have severe diarrhea, you can become dehydrated fast. Mild to moderate dehydration isn't that dangerous and can be usually corrected by drinking more fluids.

If the dehydration worsens, becomes severe, or your electrolyte levels are really out of whack, you may need to have IV fluids to correct the condition. This would require a trip down to see the ship's doctor.

Here are some signs and symptoms of mild to moderate dehydration:

- Having a dry mouth

- Feeling fatigued or sleepy all the time

- Having increased thirstiness

- Having a decreased urine output with urine that is dark yellow in color

- Having dry or flaky skin

- Being dizzy

- Having a headache

If the dehydration is allowed to worsen and you continue to lose body water, you may see the additional signs and symptoms:

- A severe reduction in the output of urine or the absence of urine at all. If there is any urine produced, it will be scant in amount and a deep yellow color or amber/brown color.

- Lightheadedness or severe dizziness that is worse when you stand up or get up from a reclining position.

- A severe drop in blood pressure that occurs when you try to get up after sitting or lying down.

- Rapid heart rate from the heart trying to compensate for a low blood volume.

- Fever, which is usually low grade in nature

- Seizures, which are usually grand mal seizures

- Poor elasticity of the skin. When you pinch it, the skin tents up and doesn't go back to its normal position.

- Being lethargic or confused

- Going into a coma

- Suffering from extreme shock, which can be life threatening.

Dehydration has a way of sneaking up on you, especially if you are otherwise occupied with other things, such as the activity you are doing or are wrapped up in being sick with vomiting and diarrhea.

As soon as you start to feel the symptoms, you need to be thinking about hydrating yourself.

Treating Mild To Moderate Dehydration

If the symptoms are mild and you can still drink, try to step up the amount of fluids you are taking in. Water is perhaps the best choice for treating dehydration. Other good choices include something like Gatorade or PowerAde, which provide liquids plus electrolytes, which can be lost in sweating, vomiting, or having diarrhea.

Over the counter anti-diarrheal medication is another choice as long as the diarrhea isn't from food poisoning. (In such cases, it is best to replace fluids only and allow the bacteria causing the diarrhea to flush out of your system). Over-the-counter medications can usually be purchased from the ships store in small packets. Prescription meds require issuance by medical staff from the ship's pharmacy.

Treating Severe Dehydration

If the dehydration is severe and you are suffering from some of the severe dehydration symptoms listed earlier, you need to consider seeing the ship's doctor and start on IV fluids.

These not only contain the water you need, but also sugar, salt and other electrolytes in solution that will restore your normal electrolyte balance. It can take as little as a liter of fluid to turn around the dehydration or as many as five or more liters depending on the severity.

Consequences Of Severe Dehydration

Besides seizures, one of the main consequences of severe dehydration includes damage to the kidneys. If the kidneys do not have fluid to flush through the tubules, you can actually suffer from acute kidney failure.

The kidneys can shut down and will only return to normal functioning with careful replacement of fluids and time. Replacing the fluids too fast, however, can result in cerebral edema and electrolyte disturbance within the brain.

Stay Hydrated

To avoid these horrible consequences, drink water regularly. While it is easy on a cruise ship, as all the bars offer free glasses of water, we don't always think about it or are more interested in drinking the "drink of the day". One trick used by veterans cruisers is to bring on empty reusable water bottle with you and then just keep refilling it. Some of the newer insulated ones will keep water cold for a long time.

Not only will you always have water to drink while on board, but also have "good" water to bring with you when off the ship on shore excursions.

Exercising

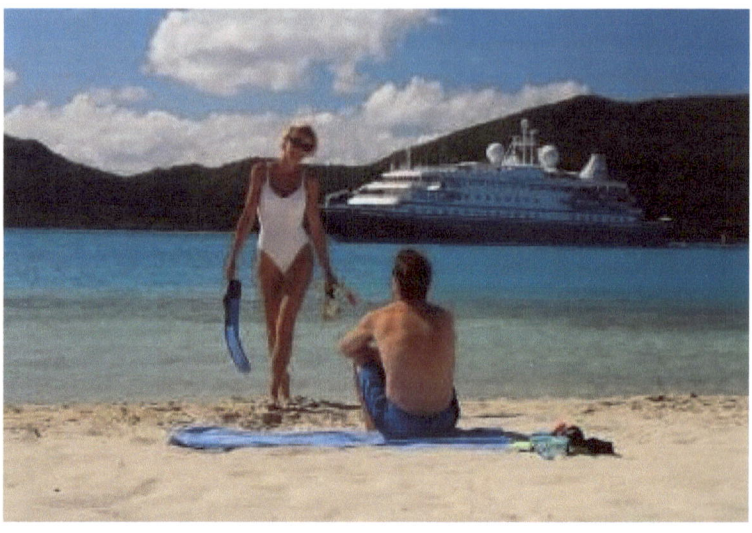

Most cruise ships today offer a well-equipped fitness center and have multiple exercise classes, climbing walls/ sports deck, etc. on board, so there isn't a reason not to get exercise. The fitness centers onboard rival anything you'll find in your hometown gym … and they are free to use. Just be sure to pick a time of day when you can get on your favorite machine without having to wait long. Usually mornings and at-sea days are when the center is the busiest. Early morning or right before mealtimes can be good times to go. The ship's fitness center is usually located close to the spa area on many ships; some centers overlook the front of the ship so you can watch what is up ahead while working out or watch the monitors on your treadmill while walking or running.

If you like group exercise classes, most ships offer yoga, Pilates, Zumba or other types of exercise classes. Most of these are also free depending on the cruise company.

If not, a nominal fee will be charged per class; you can pay with your cruise card, just like with everything else on board. There isn't a need (nor do I recommend) to carry money on your person while on board. However be sure to bring money or a credit card with you when off the ship, along with your room key card and a photo ID. In some places, you may need to bring your passport instead of an ID.

To see what kind of exercise classes are being offered during the next day, just look at your daily ship newsletter for the time and place. Show up and be prepared to work out.

Depending on your ship, it might have a sports deck that has a basketball/volleyball court or rock climbing wall. One ship we were on had a three-lane bowling alley! That could be interesting on rough sea days.

If nothing else just walk around an outside deck. Most ships even have walking or jogging paths, making it easy to get exercise. You just must get off your butt and do it.

Or exercise in the comfort of your cabin. Pack a set of resistance bands of varying strengths; they weigh almost nothing and take up little room. Do squats, lunges (both with or without resistance), push-ups and crunches right in your cabin. If you have a favorite exercise program on DVD, take it with you on your cruise and exercise to it while playing it on your computer.

Another easy way to get in steps is to take the stairs instead of the elevator. If you are only going up or down a few decks, hoof it instead of riding. It will be better for you health-wise and in many cases faster than waiting for an elevator.

In port, choose shore excursions that have you active. While it may be nice to sit on a motor coach while the tour guide explains the sights going by, or lay on a beach, you'll get more exercise if you book a shore excursion that involves exercise – like hiking, snorkeling, diving, kayaking or even exploring a town by foot; anything that will keep you moving while on land.

Eating Healthy

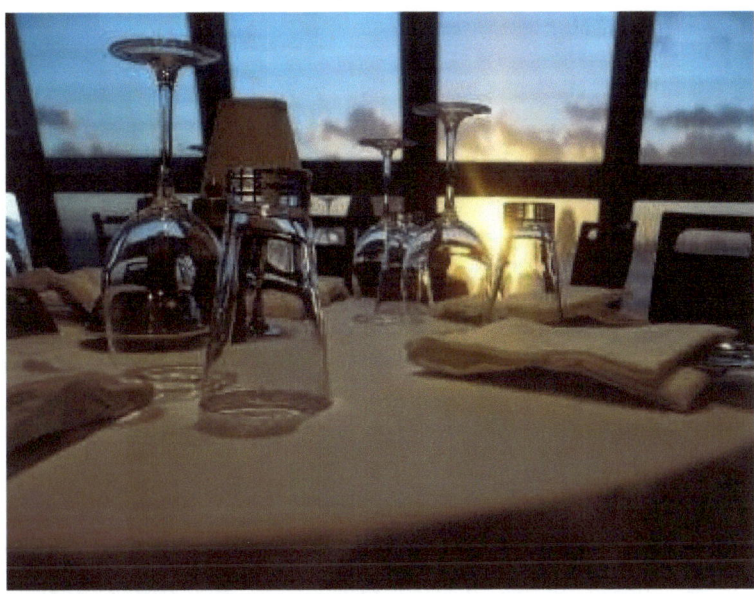

Just because cruise ships have a well-deserved reputation of having non-stop food available 24 hours a day, doesn't mean you should do your part and eat as much as you can. In excess. much of it is not good for you, such as the some of the pizza, creamy pastas and unlimited self-serve ice cream. But most cruise lines also have lighter and healthier options with less fat, sugar, salt and carbs, if you choose to be good and eat somewhat healthy.

While most of the major cruise lines have eliminated trans fat from their food fare, saturated fat is still high in many dishes. However, from their dining rooms to their buffets, most ships offer vegetarian and healthier options.

The buffet is always a good choice as they always have salad and a variety of toppings and condiments. Just watch what type of dressing you put on top.

Vinegar and oil or one of the "lighter" offerings are usually good choices.

Breakfast

Strive to eat a balance of whole grain, protein and a "good" fat for breakfast. The good fats are the unsaturated ones like olive oil. Eggs are a good choice for protein; scrambled or as part of a veggie omelet are always good choices. Oatmeal or toast are good whole grain options. If you have oatmeal, add some nuts or fruit on top with some skim or 1% milk and you have a great healthy breakfast.

Lunch

The salad bar on the buffet on most ships is a great choice for lunch. Whether you want salad to be your main entrée or as a side dish, paired with some meat for protein, is your choice. Some ships have panini grills on board, so you can get a sandwich made to order and grilled.

Dinner

The evening meals on board are not huge. On one side of the menu will be four or five offerings that are available every night. These are usually basic and appeal to a large number of people. On the other side will be the unique offerings available only on that night. Each night they change, so you get a good variety of food during the course of a cruise. If you can't find anything you like on the changeable part of the menu, you can always go with one of the non-changing offerings or go to the buffet or one of the other food venues. Some charge a nominal fee per person such as $20.00. Others will be free and included in the price of your cruise.

Want to get some exercise? Walk down to your assigned dining room mid-day to see what is on the menu for that night. It is always posted outside the dining room. You can also view the menu on the TV in your cabin (depending on the cruise line), but then you wouldn't get the exercise part in.

The big thing with eating healthy on a cruise is to eat slow and enjoy your food, so your brain has time to tell you that you are full and to stop eating. The cruise lines do a good job of helping you at dinner with this as there is usually a good block of time between courses. Plan on dinner taking about an hour to an hour and a half. With the other meals, you are on your own as far as eating slowly.

One good rule to follow is don't deny yourself anything that you want to eat. It doesn't mean you have to eat the whole thing. Take a few bites to satisfy your craving and then stop.

So whether you are home or away on vacation, here are a few good takeaways when it comes to eating:

- Indulge when it's worth it and you are really in the mood to, not just because you can or it's there
- Enjoy what you are eating/drinking – savor it and eat/drink slowly
- Pay attention to fullness cues, stopping when you are satisfied, not stuffed
- Load up on veggies when you can; they are filling and contain few calories
- Don't feel guilty for indulging in dessert if you've decided it's worth it

By using a little common eating sense, it is doubtful you would gain over a few pounds while on a week cruise. If you are good and exercise, you might not even gain anything.

It all comes down to choices and the ones you can live with without feeling guilty.

Look at the overall calories consumed during a full day. If you overindulge at one meal, back off on the next. As with many things in life, moderation is the key … and eating is no different. Don't deny yourself anything, but don't try to eat everything in sight either.

Reducing Stress

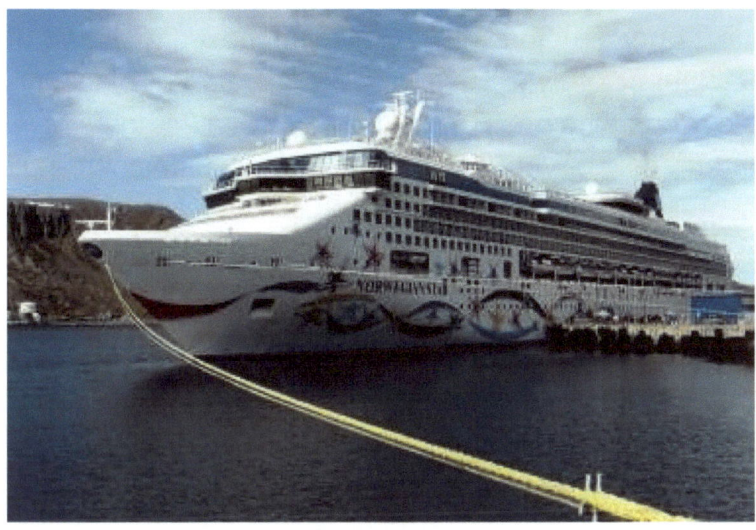

If you are within driving distance from your point of embarkation, consider yourself lucky. While even driving can be stressful, depending on weather and traffic, increased airport security, full planes, narrower seats, fewer flights to choose from and other factors have made air travel even more stressful in recent years. But in many cases, it is a necessary part of the journey getting from Point A to Point B and you just have to deal with it the best you can. With that said, however, there are things you can do to make even that mode of travel as enjoyable as possible.

Planning ahead and packing smart

These are the two best things you can do when getting ready to fly. Times for departing and incoming flights are always changing. Weather, mechanical problems, the crew showing up late, and even cancelled flights themselves, can all lead to unexpected changes.

Planning Ahead

Stay abreast of delays by checking your airline's flight status online 24 hours before your flight is supposed to depart and again right before you leave to go to the airport. Also, print out your boarding pass once you are within 24 hours of your departure time of your flight. This will save time checking in at the airport. Many times you can use one of the airline kiosk machines to check in, print out your luggage tag, drop off your luggage with an agent and you are done. Then all you must do is get through security and walk to your departing gate.

Allowing yourself ample time before your flight (two hours for domestic and three for international) can reduce some of the stress of finding parking, checking bags, moving through security, and other aspects of travel that become much more stressful when you're rushed for time. By being early, you can read a book, listen to music, or take a walk through the airport to get some exercise before you leave. Or just watching people is always fun; especially the ones that are running to catch their flight because they did not plan ahead or their first flight ran late and they are trying to make their connecting flight!

And by getting there early, if you get held up in the process of getting to your plane, at least you won't get stressed out worrying if you are going to miss your flight or not.

However, stay aware of last minute changes. Gate numbers can change for a flight while you are waiting in the boarding area. Even flights can change terminals (yes I have had that personally happen). We were at the departing gate at one terminal. It was getting to be less than an hour before boarding and there wasn't many people around.

Upon finding a monitor with departure information, the flight had not only changed to a different gate, but to a different terminal. Thankfully, the airport had an underground subway system and we got to the new gate just as they were in the middle of the boarding process.

On another trip, Dallas was iced-in and our airline kept cancelling our flight only to assign another one, but still routing us through their Dallas hub. After three changes, I (finally) got to the counter with the rest of the hoard and was told that we wouldn't get out now until Sunday (and this was on Friday).

We had a cruise to catch on Saturday. We went across the aisle and booked on an airline that went through Atlanta which was not iced-in and made our cruise in time. Once back home we requested a refund from the first airline. We finally received it after 11 months! We had all but given up hope on that refund.

Packing Smart

You can save yourself significant stress by packing wisely for your trip. Make a checklist ahead of time of all the things you need to bring with you, and check them off as you pack them to better ensure that you don't leave behind things you'll need. Pack the night before you leave, or earlier, to avoid the stress of being rushed and to give yourself the opportunity to remember and pack things you may otherwise forget (that were not on your checklist). Alternately instead of creating your own checklist from scratch, you can download one off of the Internet and modify it to fit your needs.

Keep things you may need while in transit at the ready in your carry-on bag. Passport, boarding pass, other travel documents, your phone, medications, credit cards, money, car keys and camera should always be with you. Don't pack any valuables in your check baggage – the bags that will not be in your direct control the whole time. Stow the rest of your items in your checked luggage to reduce your chances of getting slowed down at the security points.

Remember the TSA carryon policy of 3-1-1 when it comes to liquids. It stands for liquids in containers of **3** ounces or less, in a **1**-gallon plastic zip-lock bag with **1** zip-lock bag per person. With your carryon liquids in one place, you can grab it quickly and put it on the x-ray belt without holding up others behind you.

We even keep a change of clothes with us in our carryon luggage in case our checked luggage gets lost for a day or two. We do this because this has happened to us a couple of times.

It is not as bad if your luggage gets lost or delayed on the way home, but it is disconcerting if it gets lost at the start of your travel.

Dress For Comfort

While passengers used to dress up for flights in days past, we now know how important it is to dress for comfort when traveling. Be sure you wear comfortable shoes (for rushing through the airport and walking to and from your car, which may need to be parked far away). Also, be sure to wear clothes that you can comfortably move in and don't mind wearing all day.

Wear layers if you're traveling somewhere that has a cold climate; it may be cold when you leave home, cool on the airplane, but warm once you arrive at your destination. Leveryone else arouayering is the best of both worlds. Pack your carryon for the worse-case scenario and then remove and add layers as needed as the temperature rises and falls.

When you know you are going to go through airport security, leave your bling packed away in your carryon. The more jewelry you are wearing, the more stuff you will have to take off, thus slowing down the security line. Slip-on shoes are preferable to those with laces. Prepare ahead of time by removing your watch, necklace, bracelets, belt – anything that will set off the security screening machine. If you missed something, you'll just have go back, remove the item and go through again ... thus holding up those behind you. Make it easy on yourself and those around you. Think ahead and dress smart.

Note, according to TSA rules, people under the age of 12 and over the age of 75 do not have to remove their shoes. Those that have TSA PreCheck or are members of any other Global Entry program go through a special line and don't have to remove anything or take liquids or laptops out of their carryon.

Sleeping Well

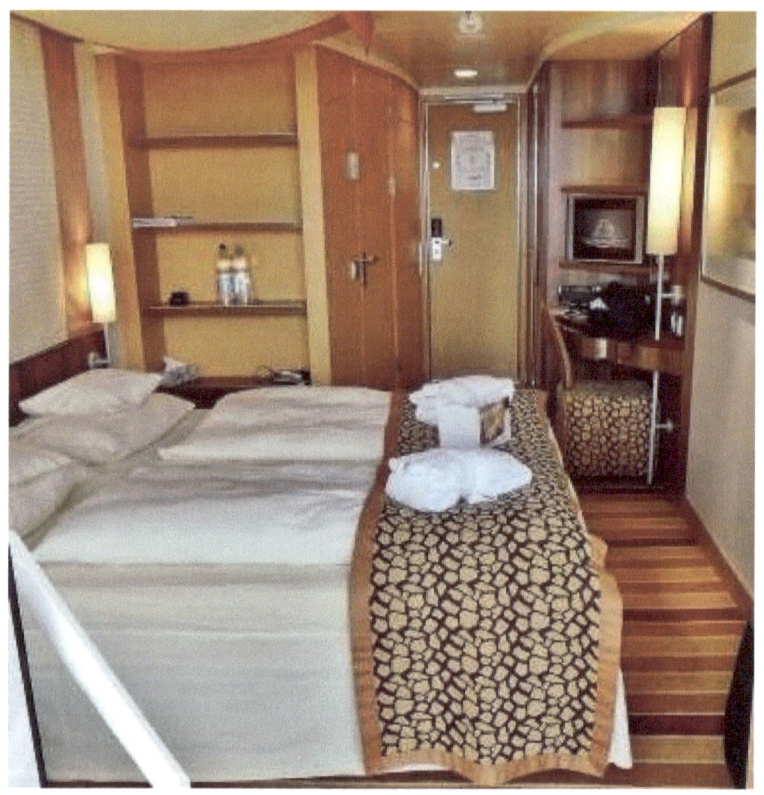

Humans are not machines and we don't keep going without breaks, although you'll see some people on a cruise try to do that. Sleep is our body's time to recharge our battery. Bottom line is sleep is essential to our health and well-being. As noted at the beginning of this book, it is one of the big three that can bring you down.

Sleep study after sleep study shows shocking evidence of the physical and mental effects of even minor levels of sleep loss and a wide range of health conditions that result from sleep deprivation.

For these reasons, it's critical that cruisers get plenty of sleep before, during and after their trips – to avoid some very critical and dangerous mistakes that can cost them their health or even their lives.

But how much is enough?

While everyone is different, WebMD, recognizes the amount of sleep a person needs depends on a number of factors, but in general the amount is determined in part by their age group:

- Infants - about 16 hours a day

- Toddlers - between 12 and 14

- Kids - between 10 and 12 hours a day

- Teenagers - about 9 hours each day

- Most adults - 7 to 8 hours a day although some need as little as 5 or as many as 10

Studies have revealed that sleep disorders cause many problems are directly tied to sleep deprivation. Here are six reasons to get the correct amount of sleep you require:

1. Memory problems

The body's ability to sleep plays a critical role in your cognitive ability – that is your ability to think and to process information.

During sleep, while the body rests, the brain is busy processing information from the day and forming memories.

Sleep is essential to the cognitive functions of the brain, and without it, our ability to consolidate memories, learn daily tasks, and make decisions is impaired.

Memory problems on your trip can mean lost luggage, missed connections, and an inability to find your hotel. Unfortunately, travel insurance isn't likely to be able to help you if the loss you're experiencing is because you forgot.

2. Weakened immune systems

It turns out that the "old wives" tale' that if you didn't sleep well, you would get sick is essentially true.

Physicians now know sleep deprivation can increase our risk of getting sick, and when prolonged, has long been associated with diminished immune functions, leaving us more prone to catching colds, the flu, and everything else in between. Sleep loss also influences our body's ability to fight an illness once it sets in.

Think about that when the guy in the next seat sneezes or coughs! Getting sick when you're traveling can make things very difficult for the rest of your trip.

3. Increased stress levels

It's been a long time since air travel was fun – everything is overcrowded, the perks are few and far between, and well, let's be honest, no one likes the TSA … although they serve an important function.

When you add the stress of travel to the increased stress on your body that results from lack of sleep, you essentially get the cortisol double-whammy.

Super high levels of cortisol in your system that result from the lack of sleep drives up anxiety levels which places greater than average stress on the body.

You might be fine as long as everything goes perfectly on your trip and you can tumble into a comfortable bed when you arrive and catch up on your sleep, but there are no such guarantees.

4. Slowed reflexes

Sleep deprivation induces significant reductions in physical performance, including reflexes and fine motor skills. This can lead to making poor decisions as noted in the next paragraph. Most of the time, the people you hear about that went overboard, made a bad decision along the way; they just did not "accidently" fall overboard. The ships are constructed in a way that with normal diligence, it is almost impossible to fall over the side. Mental impairment is usually the cause of their bad judgement, although some have went over the side intentionally thus committing suicide.

5. Poor judgement

Turns out, a lack of sleep can affect our interpretation of events. Essentially, those who are sleep-deprived do not make sound judgments because they cannot accurately assess the situation and act wisely.

Ironically, people who are running on little sleep seem to be especially prone to poor judgement when it comes to assessing how their lack of sleep is affecting them.

Excessive sleepiness also contributes to a greater risk of sustaining an injury. Mix sleep deprivation, and too much alcohol, and you have a recipe for making bad decisions and a recipe for disaster. Bad judgment is often noted as the cause for people falling overboard. That doesn't happen by accident. There is usually some bad judgement along the way leading up to the event.

Final Thoughts

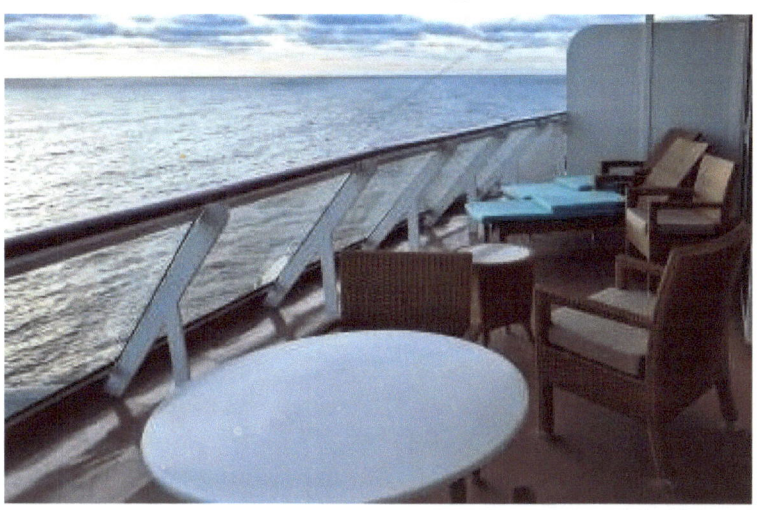

Despite doing everything right, some people still get sick. Don't trust that everyone will fill out their Public Health Questionnaire truthfully. Do you think for a minute someone that has went through the trouble to pack and travel to the port ot embarkation will mark "YES" on their form that they have been vomiting or developed symptoms of diarrhea within the last three days, or if they have had a fever and also have had one of the following: cough, runny nose or sore throat, will take a chance of not getting on board? If so, you have more faith in humanity than I do!

As soon as you mark Yes in any box, you have to be seen by the ship medical staff and evaluated to see if you are a health risk or not. If found to be one, they will deny you boarding. Most people without obvious exterior signs will simply mark "No" on their form. But because you will be among these people that were not truthful on their form, there are some things you can do to minimize the chances of getting what they have.

Wash Your Hands Frequently

Because the norovirus is always a concern when on board, the CDC recommends the best way to prevention is by washing your hands frequently with soap and hot water for at least 20 seconds. Also be sure to use the hand sanitizer stations usually posted in front of all the dining venues.

One woman posed an interesting thought: wash your hands with a 60% alcohol or greater personal hand sanitizer **after** getting your food **but** before eating – even after sanitizing your hands when coming into the area. Especially if you are eating at the buffet at the time. You never know what kind of germs the person (or people) before you had while handling the serving utensils – the same ones you used to dish up your food.

With Unclean Hands, Refrain From Touching Your Eyes, Nose or Mouth

These three places on your body are the easiest for viruses to get into your body. By refraining from touching these body parts with unclean hands as much as possible, you'll cut down on your chances of picking up something that could ruin the pleasure of your cruise.

Building Up Your Immune System

Our health professional recommends taking the immune booster Airborne three days before taking a flight, during duration of the cruise and again on the flight home. We have used this theory for the last two vacations we've taken and it seems to work for us. Taking extra vitamin C doesn't hurt anything either.

By eating right, getting enough sleep, exercising daily, taking your travel supplement routine, and frequent washing your hands, you can greatly reduce your chances of getting sick while traveling.

Make sure your vaccines are up-to-date

Make sure your normal run-of-the-mill vaccines, such as mumps, rubella, flu and chickenpox/shingles are up to date, along with any specific vaccines you may need for the area on your itinerary. Bring it to your doctor and ask if anything special is needed. On one trip into Central America for example, I had to get vaccinated for yellow fever and malaria. It is better to be safe rather than sorry later.

Take Necessary Precautions While in Port

In certain parts of the world, extra precaution might need to be taken. As of this writing, the Zika virus was active, so you might need to have insect repellant with you if traveling to an area where it is present and wear long sleeved shirts and pants to minimize the chances of getting bitten.

In many ports of call and surrounding areas, you don't want to drink the water. As mentioned earlier, fill your reusable water bottle or buy bottled water on board before getting off of the ship.

Travel Insurance

When we were younger (and thought we were invincible) we never purchased travel insurance. Now that we are older (and wiser), and after reading about some of the horror stories of getting sick while traveling, we now buy it on every cruise.

For us it runs about $100 each for a week's cruise, but that is cheap. The price is determined by your age and duration of your cruise.

If you have to be medevac'd off of the ship while at sea for example, it can run as high as $50,000. All of a sudden, that $100 you paid for insurance looks really cheap. And it can cover you for other things too, such as missing your cruise due to flight delays or cancellations, if you get sick at home and can't make your cruise, etc. Like all insurance, it is better to have it and not need it rather than to need it and not have it.

That about does it as far as staying healthy while on a cruise. As you gain more experience with this fantastic method of traveling, you'll also develop your own methods of staying well. But in the meantime, the tips and techniques in this book should help you get started and stay healthy on your first cruise.

Other Relevant Books by This Author

If you would like to read more about Senior Health and Fitness, here is a list of the titles, CreateSpace links and descriptions:

https://www.createspace.com/3859041

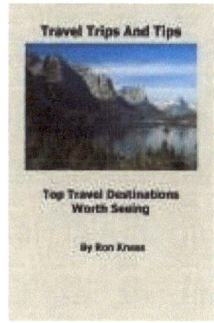

Travel Trips and Tips

The destinations in this guide are either places I have personally already visited (some several times each) or ones I have thoroughly researched and are on my bucket list to see. I wanted to deviate from traditional travel guides in that these are my personal experiences and research.

https://www.createspace.com/4962939

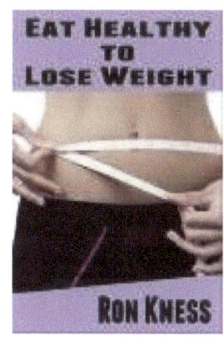

Eat Healthy to Lose Weight

As you read through our book, we show you which foods you should and should not be eating to reach your weight loss goal, along with discussing how to maintain your weight loss and stay within a few pounds of your goal weight. Banish the weight you keep gaining back each time by learning how to live a healthy lifestyle.

https://www.createspace.com/5416348

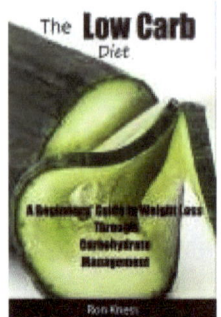

The Low Carb Diet: A Beginner's Guide to Weight Loss Through Carbohydrate Management

In my book "The Low-Carb Diet – A Beginners' Guide to Weight Loss Through Carbohydrate Management", I reveal a successful method of losing weight based in part on the amount and type of carbohydrates you consume. This healthy way of eating works and doesn't leave you feeling hungry.

https://www.createspace.com/6365965

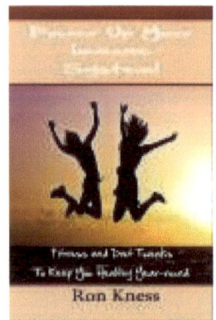

Power Up Your Immune System!

Do you seem to catch colds or the flu easily?

Are you resigned to the fact that you are just "one of those people" that is naturally prone to infection and illness? Maybe you regularly plan for getting sick a few times each year when the seasons change. Guess what? Your family tree and genetic makeup deserve only a small amount of influence over your immune system.

That means it is possible to give your body's natural level of immunity a boost. You really can start fighting off unhealthy and dangerous bacteria, viruses and germs, simply by making some lifestyle changes.

And this is true whether you are young or old, male or female, and regardless where you live in the world.

In this book, we explore some fitness and diet adjustments you can make that can power up your immune system, thus keeping you healthier year-round.

About the Author

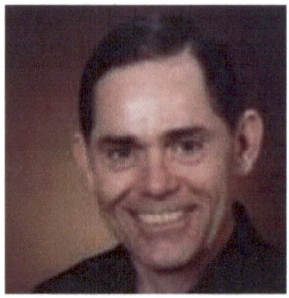

I grew up in Central Minnesota, where my parents owned and operated a fishing resort. Once out of high school I tried a couple of semesters of college, only to quit halfway through the Spring term; I decided at that time that college wasn't for me.

Then I decided to follow my father's previous occupation as an auto mechanic. I graduated from a two-year of vocational training course and worked as a mechanic for five years. While in vocational training, I decided to join the National Guard where I eventually ended up working full-time for 32 years.

So how does all of this relate to writing? In one of my leadership schools, the instructor, who was an English teacher at a juvenile detention center, presented writing to me in a whole new way - a way that started to develop my interest in working with words.

I eventually went back to college on the GI Bill while I was working and earned my Bachelor's degree in Business Administration. Taking a class or two per semester at night and on weekends took me seven years to complete my degree.

Fast forward about 40 years and I now have published over 75 books on Amazon for Kindle, CreateSpace and other publishing platforms.

Besides my own writing, I also ghostwrite ebooks, reports, articles, blogs and do Kindle conversions for clients on a variety of topics.

Today my wife and I are retired from our careers and live in Gold Canyon, AZ. I now write as a retirement business where you'll find me happily sitting in my office typing away on my laptop as I work on my next book or ghostwriting project . . . that is if we are not traveling on a cruise ship - our new-found mode of travel.

www.ingramcontent.com/pod-product-compliance
Lightning Source LLC
Chambersburg PA
CBHW040316010626
45792CB00022B/640